AM I TOO OLD FOR A MILLION DOLLAR SMILE?

A CONSUMERS GUIDE TO COMPREHENSIVE DENTAL TREATMENT FOR ADULTS

BEHZAD NAZARI, DDS

Camva Publishing Company

Am I Too Old For A Million Dollar Smile?
A Consumers Guide To Comprehensive Dental Treatment For Adults
Copyright © 2017 Behzad Nazari, DDS

Camva Publishing Company
701 E. Burress
Houston, Texas 77022

Book design by:
Arbor Books, Inc.
www.arborservices.co/

Printed in the United States of America

Am I Too Old For A Million Dollar Smile?
A Consumers Guide To Comprehensive Dental Treatment For Adults
Behzad Nazari, DDS

1. Title 2. Author 3. Dentistry

Library of Congress Control Number: 2017901988
ISBN 13: 978-0-692-84485-4

Contents

Introduction

When a loved one is ill, it hits home with a stark reality; over twenty years ago my father suffered a major heart attack, and my family faced a challenge that they had never experienced. As a dentist, one of these challenges involved me directly taking care of my father's dental needs.

I am happy to say my father survived his heart attack, and as I sit here writing this, he is alive and well. During his recovery, though, not only did I come to appreciate this wonderful man even more than I ever had before (and I have always appreciated and loved my dad), but I began to see my work in a completely different way.

It's fairly routine for a dentist to treat the adult patient coming in for a regular cleaning or one with no health complications needing to replace a missing tooth with an implant. But when you consider an adult patient like my father dealing with a specific health problem and taking several medications for it, the complications from and for dental treatment can become life threatening. For instance, how often do we consider our teeth and gums when we take medicine for a condition that has nothing whatsoever to do with our dental health? Or how about the adult patient who may have undergone some specific drug treatment or surgery decades before, how often do we consider the lasting effects of these medicines and procedures when they come in for dental procedures in the present? And unless warned by our doctor, would a patient ever really know when a seemingly routine dental procedure might affect their compromised health?

Exploring the options for my father's dental visits post heart attack, gaining a clearer view of adult dental care in general, I came to recognize a great reluctance from adult patients to receive comprehensive dental treatment. The majority choose what I call "patch-up" dentistry. A few comments we dentists commonly hear are: "Just take care of this tooth, Doc, I am too old for all that work." "It does not bother me now; I'll come back when it hurts." "Root canal? No thanks, Doc. Just pull it." I quickly realized that adult patients hardly ever address the root of their mouth's problems when they go in for this à la carte dental care.

Surely fear, expense, and time are more reasons—and often the primary reasons—for adults to ignore comprehensive dental treatment, but also a patient's apathetic attitude toward dentistry is another reason he or she might not pursue better dental care. Dental health simply becomes something many adults don't care so much about as they get older; they simply learn to live with what bothers them. Their mouth has been in pain or their chewing uncomfortable for so long anyway, why address it now?

But time and again I have seen all these reasons and more fall away once a patient becomes interested in having a new smile. The promise of a healthy-looking big pearly white grin pushes many an adult patient beyond their fears and assumptions. I have seen this happen so many times I have lost count!

Sure, lots of adult patients simply think they are too old to get the smile of their dreams. They believe what they have is all they can get. They believe notions such as: "Bad teeth run in my family" or "I've got my mother's teeth; she lost all her teeth in her thirties after her third child" or "We all have bad enamel; my brother and sister have partials." Or one I often hear: "But after root canals, don't teeth crumble? Why should I save them if they crumble?" My father had this negative view after his recovery, even though I'm a dentist and he knew I would do all in my power to make his teeth as healthy as I could. He told me on several occasions: "My days are numbered. What's the point of getting all this work done?" "My father always used wet paper towels to reline and stabilize his dentures. He lived like that, and I can do it, too." "Implants are not for me."

Luckily, I convinced my father that we could take care of his dental work, and he agreed to go in for a smile makeover. He now flashes his beautiful teeth every chance he gets, his dentures and implants fit perfectly, and his chewing has never been better. He now smiles with confidence, like so many of my adult patients who thought they never would. He is not embarrassed any longer about showing his teeth, and in fact, my father was such an inspiration with his newfound smile—and wonderful attitude from it—when my mother saw how fantastic my dad's outcome was, she decided to get a smile makeover too!

My father's cardiologist also had an interest in my father's improved dental health. In working to see my father fully recovered, his doctor impressed upon us the benefits of better nutrition, and to have better nutrition, my father needed to have better teeth to chew his food. God knows my dad does love his food, from shish kabobs to crawfish, and now he can chew those foods he loves rather than just bite and swallow them. Even foods that were so hard for him to eat before—many foods the cardiologist truly wanted to get into my father's diet—are now possible for my father to eat . . . and enjoy.

This new life attitude from a smile is not exclusive to my father or to a few patients. Many middle-aged and older adult men and women think like this. Every day, dentists in good faith sit face-to-face with their adult patients to present comprehensive treatment plans, explaining to them that they are not too old, that they deserve optimum oral health and can surely have a million-dollar smile.

In the end, it is much easier to overcome fear and money-related issues than it is to change one's mental attitude about dental care. By no means am I underplaying the fear of dentistry or the high cost of major dental treatment; however, I am pointing out the reality that fear and money are not the only barriers for patients accepting dental treatment.

This book is intended to address the concerns that adult patients have when it comes to their teeth and smile. I will try and answer common questions reluctant men and women have about dental treatment, explore the many options of modern dentistry, and hope to introduce you all to the real possibility of having, once and for all, the million-dollar smile.

The ultimate goal of any dental care provider is to restore and maintain health to the patient's dentition and oral cavity as a whole, for life. And the more consistent a patient is in seeing their dentist, the better that dental care will be. For all intents and purposes, dentistry should be viewed as a preventive discipline. Regular visits to a dentist serve to detect and prevent decay and periodontal disease, address gum disease in its early stages, and stop tooth decay from progressing. Simple restorations can help a patient avoid complicated procedures. And even root canals prevent tooth loss, and implants prevent bone loss, which in turn will prevent major impairment to the masticatory (chewing) system. All these procedures increase the odds for a properly functioning mouth and the patient's ability to receive the best nutrition. And at the same time, your dentist will make your smile better, more beautiful and pleasing.

Modern dentistry assures that the adult patient can have healthy, properly functioning teeth and a great-looking smile.

Really, what could be better than that?

CHAPTER 1

The Smile:
A Brief History of Why It's So
Important

Imagine how much more famous Mona Lisa would be if she had said "cheese" while posing for Leonardo da Vinci. Teeth and smiles have always had a special value for us. Even as babies we realize how much we can gain just by smiling at whoever is paying attention to us.

The gesture of a smile is not a recent phenomenon. Smiling has been traced back thirty million years. A primatologist, Signe Preuschoft, found the "fear grin" in primates, where early apes revealed their harmlessness to predators by smiling at them. Later on in a famous scientific study, French Neurologist Guillaume Duchenne put his name to the two types of smiles we humans show. The Duchenne smile is an organic spontaneous smile, a reaction to any number of positive stimuli, where both the muscles of the eyes and mouth come into play, a sign of enjoyment. The non-Duchenne smile is where we only use our mouth to smile; it's that fake "say cheese" smile we have all painted across our faces from time to time. Each one reveals the smiler's teeth, so there is no getting around the fact that the nicer your teeth are, the nicer your smile will be.

Charles Darwin, who corresponded with Duchenne and used the French man's illustrations in one of his books, studied nonverbal body language and learned when doing so that babies begin smiling at five weeks. This led Darwin to conclude further that we are set through our DNA to connect with our fellows by smiling at, and with, them. It's no wonder then that psychologists have found that people who cannot or do not smile have more difficulty socializing with others.

Yes, we might be used to seeing celebrities flashing impossibly bright smiles we know are the result of some dentist working his or her magic, but believe it or not, cosmetic dentistry is not a new phenomenon. Throughout history men and women have tried to bring attention to themselves through their smile by various means, as teeth aesthetics have been a priority for humans since the dawn of civilization. Cosmetic dental procedures have been practiced in one form or another for several thousand years, with some archeologists estimating those procedures dating as far back as nine thousand years! In Egyptian excavations, archeologists have found beautifully carved teeth made from shells in jaw bones, indicating that these shells were early implants used to replace missing teeth. Mayan excavations have revealed decorated teeth with pieces of jade and other jewelry drilled into a skeleton's teeth. Were these hip-hop stars of their day? And well-to-do Etruscan ladies (circa 800–200 BC) would have their front teeth removed so that goldsmiths could fit them with a gold band to hold their replacement teeth in their mouths.

We are lost without our smiles. Not smiling, or covering our mouth with our hand every time we experience the urge to flash the spontaneous

Duchenne smile, becomes a habit over time, but it sure takes its toll on one's psyche. In no time at all, people set their mood to the fact that they don't want to or are afraid to smile. We see people like this all the time, don't we? Keeping their heads down, avoiding contact, letting the fact that they hate their smile make them more ill-tempered and morose. Might this be you, going through life with no hope that you'll ever smile again?

Don't worry. Your smile is still there. Together you and your dentist can help you join the social world again.

There is proof from leading scientists, anthropologists, physicians, psychologists, and years of historical record that smiling provides benefits beyond just the aesthetic. Yes, Julia Roberts and Denzel Washington might be known for their smiles, and you might very well envy them for it, but scientific fact backs up the claim that smiling can go a long way toward making you feel better. Smiling has been shown to release dopamine, endorphins, and serotonin. These chemicals relax the body overall, act as natural pain suppressors, and lower heart rate and blood pressure.

So you see, smiling is good for your body as well as your spirit.

Your smile isn't gone for good. Your life will improve; you will feel young again. You will be able to maintain strong and healthy white rows of teeth. What you had once years ago or maybe what you have only ever dreamed about is possible. It is out there; your smile is waiting for you. As we will see, modern adult dentistry is the best it has ever been (all healthcare, in fact, is the best it has ever been) and those men and women who have given up on ever smiling, for whatever reason, now have hope to smile again.

The million-dollar smile is all about how your smile makes you feel. It's not limited to just Hollywood smiles of pearly white, perfectly shaped straight teeth. Any improvement in your smile that makes you feel like a million bucks is your million-dollar smile. The answer to the title of this book "Am I too old for a million-dollar smile?" is a resounding NO.

CHAPTER 2

Living Longer . . . While Keeping
Those Teeth in Your Head

Good dental hygiene, a consistent and vigorous at-home dental regimen, and regular visits to your dentist are paramount to enjoying good dental health . . . and for keeping your million-dollar smile. The CDC (the Centers for Disease Control and Prevention, found here: http://www.cdc.gov/nccdphp/publications/CDNR/) offers these tenets for keeping your teeth as long as you can:

- Drink fluoridated water and use a fluoride toothpaste; fluoride's protection against tooth decay works for anyone of any age.
- Brush regularly and vigorously and floss daily to reduce dental plaque and prevent gingivitis—the mildest form of gum disease.
- Smokers have four times the risk of developing gum disease compared to nonsmokers. Using tobacco in any form, be it cigarettes, pipes, or chewing tobacco, increases the risk for gum disease, oral and throat cancers, and oral fungal infection (candidiasis). Spitting tobacco even contains sugar, which increases the risk of tooth decay. Teeth staining and discoloration also increase in smokers.

- Limit alcohol use. Heavy alcohol use is also a risk factor for oral and throat cancers. Combined with smoking, the effects of alcohol grow even greater. Teeth staining and discoloration also increase with excess alcohol use.

- Eat wisely. Adults should avoid snacks full of sugars and starches. Limit the number of snacks you eat throughout the day. The recommended five-a-day helping of fiber-rich fruits and vegetables stimulates salivary flow to aid remineralization of tooth surfaces that could be in the early stages of tooth decay.

- Visit the dentist regularly. Check-ups can detect early signs of oral health problems and can lead to treatments that will prevent further damage, and in some cases, reverse the problem. Professional tooth cleaning (prophylaxis) is also important for preventing oral problems, especially when self-care is difficult.

- Diabetic patients should work to maintain control of their disease. One of the many complications of diabetes is an increased risk of gum disease.

- Have an oral health check-up before beginning cancer treatment. Radiation to the head or neck, and chemotherapy may cause problems for your teeth and gums. Treating existing oral health problems before cancer therapy may help prevent or limit oral complications or tissue damage.

While increased life expectancy is certainly a wonderful result of our advances in medicine and technology, one of the big questions we face in this modern age is: how do we live longer and maintain good health while doing so? Life expectancy is presently the highest it has ever been. The average life span in 1965 was sixty-five years; it increased to seventy-eight years in 1990, and now an eighty-year-old can expect to live eight more years. All this is good news, but we need to consider that the longer a person lives, the more possible it is that stuff will wear out. As we age, our body changes, from internal organs such as kidneys, liver, and lungs, to our brain, eyes, ears, teeth, and skin—all are affected by the aging process. So we should be paying attention to our mouths as we should to all of our body.

Interestingly, adults often do not address their dental concerns for the simple reason that they are getting older, that they feel stuff wearing out. Many men and women lose interest in caring for what they feel they are destined for. Like getting wrinkles or needing thicker glasses, many adults figure that over time, their teeth are just going to go.

Adult patients also face other challenges younger ones do not:

- The side effects of certain medications the more mature person might be taking (for high blood pressure, anxiety, Parkinson's disease, and many others) might cause the patient to experience xerostomia, or dry mouth, which can lead to many dental complications.
- As with many parts of our body, enamel wears out over time, and teeth chipping and breakage become more likely as we get older. Adults also experience their gums receding, which could lead to a whole host of heretofore unrealized dental problems such as cervical caries and sensitivity to cold or hot.
- We also lose skin elasticity as we age, which can affect one's lip tone, hindering one's ability to smile and even eat properly.

Behzad Nazari, DDS

- Many adults of any age might have real concern over insurance and how they might be able to pay for their dental care.

Most of the above concerns can be addressed in a variety of ways. The adult patient need not ignore their dental health, and they don't need to ignore any other aspect of what is happening to their decidedly aging, yet still vitally alive bodies. Yes, there might be plenty wrong with your mouth. Yes, you may have let tooth decay go on far too long. You might feel guilt and shame just thinking about having to open your mouth for a dentist after all this time. Yes, you might even enjoy being the Grumpy Gus, reveling in that reputation you have of never smiling, of being unapproachable. But because of modern adult dentistry, none of the above has to be your lot in life. All studies show that you have many productive years ahead, so why not smile wide to the approaching future?

CHAPTER 3

Modern Dentistry: Art As Well As Science

Dentistry is as much an art as it is a science. Advances in diagnostic tools, dental surgery techniques, as well as new machinery and materials have decreased the amount of time procedures take while assuring longer lasting and cosmetically superior restorations by the dentist's skilled hand.

In what follows you will find the various procedures as well as the reason for your dentist proposing them, assuring you the healthiest teeth and gums, and that big, beautiful, confident smile.

Paraphrasing Shakespeare in regard to modern dentistry: "There are more things in technology and science, Horatio, than you ever dreamt of in your dentist's chair."

Following are just some of the few new advancements that you may have never dreamt of but that will certainly get you back in a dentist's chair:

Invisalign® – The word Invisalign has more or less become synonymous with modern adult braces—like the Kleenex® brand name replacing the word tissue—to the degree that these removable custom-made clear plastic aligners have brought more adults to consider braces than any other advancement in orthodontics. The number one concern of men and women wanting their teeth straight is that they simply do not want to have to walk around with a mouthful of metal at their age. With Invisalign, adult patients can have their teeth straightened by a nearly undetectable apparatus.

Dental Implants – Dental implants are artificial replacements for the tooth root. Dental implants are fabricated from titanium and look like screws. They are considered by the profession to be the best treatment for replacing a missing tooth or teeth.

We will discuss modern dental implants later in this book.

Digital X-rays – Remember those days of old when your dentist would drape a heavy lead blanket down your torso, work hard to position the nozzle of his X-ray machine to your face . . . then promptly skip out of the room? Then he'd have to try and determine what it was he saw in the shadows of the film's black and white image. This kind of diagnostic tool is a dinosaur lumbering to extinction in the face of modern digital X-ray capacity. Dentists can now take digital pictures of a patient's mouth faster, involving less radiation (about 90% less), and have the image appear on a computer screen in a matter of moments. These images are clearer and more defined than ever before, allowing the doctor to zoom in, as well as look at the X-ray from multiple angles. This advancement in technology saves both patient and dentist lots of time.

3D Cone Beam Imaging – Related to the advancement and better overall safety of digital X-rays, dentists can now study a more realistic three-dimensional view of their patients' head and neck structures through the use of a specific type of imaging software. A dentist can study, rotate, and manipulate dental measurements, a multisided view of the structure of the jaw, and the full view of a patient's craniofacial anatomy. This kind of imaging better facilitates the exact location of any nerve paths, pathology, placing implants, and surgeries.

Better Materials – Upgrades in resins, plastics, ceramics, and implants assure patients of longer-lasting prosthetics and fillings. Along with the upgrade in both the durability and malleability of these newer and better materials, greater attention has been paid to the aesthetics of restorations, making the matching of prosthetic (false) teeth color the best it has ever been.

Oral and IV Sedation – Advances in materials and procedures are one thing, but how about what a dentist can currently do to alleviate a patient's pain and anxiety while in the dental chair? As with all the above, great strides in dental anesthesia have made the patient's visit more pleasant. There are now oral and IV sedations that truly make procedures possible for all, whereas in the past, there were restrictions on who could benefit from each specific sedation. For those adults with a low pain threshold, a crippling fear of the dentist, overly sensitive teeth, or those having to undergo a significant amount of dental work, modern sedation makes visits to the dentist endurable.

These days the doses of both oral and IV sedation can vary from minimal to moderate, all safely administered through the use of modern drugs that carry the slightest amount of side effects. With IV sedation especially, sedation can be adjusted even during the procedure at the dentist's determination.

New Technology in Oral Cancer Screening – VELscope and ViziLite are examples of devices that use fluorescence technology to help dental diagnosticians identify oral cancer, precancer, and other abnormal lesions in the oral cavity. Based on a report by ADA, thirty-five thousand cases of mouth, throat, and tongue cancer are found each year, with the average age of people diagnosed being sixty-two years old.

To learn more about the rise of oral cancer, go to www.oralcancerfoundation.org for relevant articles and current data.

CAD/CAM – Computer-aided designs are used in manufacturing dental prosthetics: single unit restorations such as inlays, onlays, and crowns. The CAD/CAM restorations are highly accurate and can be fabricated immediately (same-day crowns). Another application of CAD/CAM technology is to develop surgical guides for implant placement.

CHAPTER 4

General Dental Health

In the everyday practice of dentistry, dentists encounter so many questions and concerns. We certainly understand that what we do is pretty much alchemy to the layman and for those patients who haven't been to a dentist for a long time, so many of our procedures and instrumentation might seem like apparatuses and approaches right out of *Star Trek*.

But as much as your dentist knows about treating your mouth, making your smile bigger, better, and brighter, he or she won't know about the rest of your health unless you are forthcoming about what's going on with your body presently.

Simply put, what affects the mouth affects the body, and vice versa. Your smile might be something you very much want to maintain or even get back, but also remember that beyond how pearly white and straight your teeth look, your mouth is the gateway to your body. (Don't doctors always ask us first to open wide and say, "Ahhh?").

Many nondental medical conditions and their treatment do affect the mouth, while dental procedures and the conditions of the mouth can adversely affect and compromise overall health. This is why, as we will see later, the adult dental patient's medical history is so important, especially with adults who present with past or current medical conditions and sometimes undetected systemic disease.

With advancing age comes a possible increase in chronic medical conditions and chronic prescription drug use to treat those systemic diseases, and both a disease and a drug can affect the health of the mouth. Detailed discussions of medical conditions and their significance on dentistry are beyond the scope of this book, but consider these examples:w

- The patient with good oral hygiene, brushing, flossing, and visiting the dentist regularly who still suffers from gingival overgrowth. This gingival overgrowth might be a sign of an underlying medical condition such as leukemia, or a side effect of medications to control epilepsy.

- Sudden changes in a patient's bite can result from conditions such as acromegaly (an abnormal sudden growth of hands, feet, and face caused by the pituitary gland overproducing a patient's growth hormone). The neoplasm (overgrown tissue) causes enlargement of the jaw, and conventional dental treatment might not correct the problem without first addressing the underlying medical condition.

- Cancer, chemotherapy, bleeding disorders, and anticoagulant medications can cause excessive bleeding after dental procedures, especially those that are invasive.

- Burning mouth/tongue syndrome is a sign of several medical conditions such as anemia or vitamin deficiency.

- Oral thrush can be a side effect of many antibiotics or the immuno-suppressive medications taken after kidney transplant procedures. Chemotherapy, AIDS, cancer, and diabetes are other illnesses that can inhibit the immune system and contribute to oral thrush also.
- Heartburn or GERD can lead to enamel erosion of the teeth because of the acidic nature of the mouth.
- Chronic use of antidepressants, antianxiety pills, sleeping aids, and pain management medications that are widely used in today's society almost all have oral-related side effects, notably dry mouth.
- Patients on blood thinner therapy may have bleeding complications after dental procedures such as tooth extraction or periodontal surgery.

Postmenopausal females suffering from osteoporosis and who have been on bisphosphonate therapy might sometimes suffer a classic example of the connection between the complications between medication and dental treatment. While pharmaceutical companies with all their TV and magazine advertising work hard to give the impression that medications such as bisphosphonates are safe, in fact, patients taking bisphosphonate have been known to have many jaw bone complications after dental treatments.

There is also overwhelming evidence of a relationship between periodontal and heart disease, a serious issue. Periodontal disease must be treated to reduce the chronic inflammation that contributes to cardiovascular disease. Dental treatment of patients with heart conditions such as mitral valve prolapse, heart murmurs, and joint replacement can develop life-threatening infections if not premedicated with a proper antibiotic.

The numbing medicine Lidocaine, which is widely used in dentistry, can affect a susceptible heart patient since Lidocaine is also used as anti-arrhythmic medicine. Furthermore, the amount and type of any anesthetic administered by the dentist to patients with heart disease or high blood pressure must be carefully adjusted to prevent any complications.

Antianxiety medicine, tranquilizers, and painkillers are routinely prescribed by dentists to alleviate anxiety and control pain. Many patients take the same medications or similar for medical reasons, and too much of these medications could lead to an overdose and dangerous results.

All of the above reasons—and quite a few more—are why it is important for patients to let their dentist know if there have been any changes in their health; what their overall health condition is; and to list past health concerns, procedures, and what medications they may have taken or are presently prescribed. Your dentist needs to know about your health history and needs to be able to communicate with the other medical professionals you visit on a regular basis. All the people who attend to your health want to give you the best care they can.

A dental appointment time and duration must also be taken into consideration depending on a patient's physical endurance. To work all day then drive through rush-hour traffic to get to a dental office is exhausting for a patient who already has compromised health. Early or late morning appointments and taking off work on the day of dental appointment are highly recommended. Treatment plans for these patients also need to be divided into multiple short appointments to reduce stress. IV or oral sedation in many situations is warranted.

Referral to a hospital-based dental facility should always be considered in patients with severe systemic disease to anticipate unexpected complications should they arise.

The first step in managing a patient with medical problems is to acquire a comprehensive health history through a written questionnaire and verbal interview. After a physical evaluation and dental examination, the dental clinician should consider the patient's health status and weigh it against the dental treatment before embarking on any procedures. The dental clinician must fully understand the significance of the disease stated and obtain proper medical consultation and release; after all "do no harm" is part of the Hippocratic Oath. A few patients find it inconvenient at first, but after explaining the significance and potential danger to their health, they are usually more than willing to follow through with all the recommendations.

Below are some further questions you might have about basic dental procedures. Where possible, questions have been printed verbatim to show you that your concerns are the same ones many patients have.

CHAPTER 5

Q&A:
General Dental Health

What should I expect when I go to a dentist, and how do I choose the right dentist?

At any dental office, you must complete a comprehensive medical and dental questionnaire, followed by a verbal review conducted by a member of the dental team or doctor. Then they must obtain your vital signs, which will usually include your blood pressure, heart rate, and body weight. Necessary X-rays are taken, then the doctor will conduct an oral examination, including a head and neck exam and oral cancer screening.

You must be honest and precise about your answers. Do not be shy or embarrassed; do not hide anything from your dentist. We all have some kind of medical issues. An honest dialogue must be established from the beginning.

As much as you desire to get free from pain or have radiant rows of resplendently reflecting beautiful teeth to enjoy a functional bite, your health and safety come first. Medical emergencies in dental offices are easily preventable with good communication between dentist, staff, and patient.

Do your homework. You can do extensive research about dentists on the Internet. Sophisticated treatments need a multispecialty approach. Make sure the dentist you are considering is experienced and treats middle aged and elderly patients with similar dental issues to yours or works with a network of specialists that they can refer to.

Observe other patients while in the reception area. Do you see more children or adult patients?

Remember, there is no such thing as a super dentist, no man or woman who can do everything that needs to be done in a patient's mouth. As there are optometrists, gynecologists, allergists, and dermatologists, there are dentists who specialize in specific dental health disciplines. You wouldn't trust your knee to a cardiologist, and you should not trust your implants to a dentist whose majority of patients are children.

Next, check out how the dental exam is conducted. Is there a systematic approach? Does the dentist ask the right questions to address your concerns, and are you given the opportunity to ask questions? Do you feel you have been heard, that you have been understood? Are your concerns addressed?

A more comprehensive and thorough examination of patients consists of taking a series of X-rays called a full-mouth series, and if necessary, a panoramic X-ray; visual examination of the oral cavity (the mouth), including teeth and soft and hard tissue surrounding the teeth; oral cancer screening; and even making diagnostic casts if needed. As to be expected, a more involved diagnosis and the presentation of more varied treatment options may take more than one to two appointments depending on the complexity of the case. You also need to feel out the dentist to determine if he or she is the right one for you.

I went to the dentist, and he gave me only one treatment plan option. How do I know if there is anything else that can be done?

In dentistry, usually there are several alternative treatment options. For example, a simple filling can be done with a silver amalgam, tooth color resin, or porcelain inlay/onlay . . . depending on the size of the filling; a crown might even be appropriate. If tooth loss is unavoidable, it can be replaced with an implant, bridge, or a removable partial denture.

I went to two different dentists, and their treatment plans are very different; why?

As mentioned above, there can be two or more treatment options for the same diagnosis. The training and experience of the dentist, and his or her clinical expertise will influence the treatment options recommended. For example, some dentists are comfortable placing extra-large (complex) fillings in the tooth, while other dentists are not, recommending crowns instead. Some dentists have a "wait and watch" philosophy and some do not; some dentists recommend waiting to see if incipient cavities get bigger in the future, and some dentists won't do this. Some might recommend only implants, while others may recommend bridges and removable partial dentures to replace missing teeth. Patients always have the right to a second opinion and to choose a treatment that fits their budget and what they want to have done.

My dentures make me gag. I know I have no teeth and dentures are the only option, but can you make them smaller?

You do not have to live with loose wobbly and large dentures that make you gag. Dental implants are the answer. When it comes to implants and dentures, you have two options:

Implant supported removable dentures – these are less bulky, but you still have to take them out and clean them.

Implant supported fixed dentures that you cannot remove; your dentist attaches your denture teeth permanently to implants, so they act and feel just like your natural teeth.

Do I still need to brush and floss and see my dentist for cleaning after implants?

Yes, you still have to brush and floss your implant teeth and visit your dentist regularly. Your dentist will let you know how often you need to have regular dental check-ups. You will not have cavities in the implants, of course, but the soft tissue and bone holding your implants can get infected and decrease the life span of your implants.

Why are my teeth so sensitive lately? Is this simply a sign of old age?

Yes, it can be. Over time, enamel can wear thin (this is also one of the reasons why, after some time, it might seem that your teeth appear duller), but teeth sensitivity can be caused by a few factors. You might be suffering from tooth decay, or over time your gums might have receded from your teeth a bit, exposing a tooth root surface that causes hot or cold sensitivity. Other issues that can lead to tooth sensitivity but are usually temporary can be reactions after tooth bleaching, dental treatments such as fillings, after having a tooth crowned, and deep cleaning.

Should I get all my teeth pulled? I am missing some in the back, most of my teeth have fillings in them from thirty years ago, and the teeth in front are so crooked that food keeps getting stuck between them and even with a toothpick I cannot take the meat out.

An initial comprehensive medical and dental evaluation/exam is necessary before your dentist can recommend any treatment, from the simplest cases to something as complex as the above question. As mentioned before, patients have a broad range of options these days with modern dentistry, and benefits vs. risk, long-term cost, and many other factors need to be taken into consideration.

Can you explain dental insurance? I have reams of paper and lots of terms in my coverage, but I really don't understand what's covered and what's not. Should I be looking for a better policy, and what exactly is better?

This is a complicated question . . .

Unlike medical insurances that have large dollar benefits, dental insurances do not cover much, on average anywhere from $1,000 to $2,500 per year. It usually serves the patient to take advantage of their dental insurance for preventive work, since preventive treatments are usually covered at 100% (it benefits you to study your contract's terms), but they are not helpful with complicated treatments and procedures that can run several thousands of dollars.

Dental insurance was first offered in 1850 by the Franklin Health Insurance Company of Massachusetts, introduced in California over a hundred years later, and then began its rise in popularity with the general American public. In the 1970s there were a wide variety of plans available, usually offered by the Delta Dental Company, with these plans usually offering a maximum annual coverage of $1,000, which is still generally the maximum today. These first plans did not distinguish between in-network and out-of-network providers. They simply establishing rates for a given geographic area, paying 100% for preventive care, 80% for minor dental work (fillings, etc.), and 50% for any major procedures (crowns, bridges, etc.). In a competitive capitalist marketplace, other plans began to be offered, most notably the Dental Preferred Provider Organization. A who's who list of PPO companies included Guardian Insurance, Blue Cross Blue Shield, United Health-care, Concordia, MetLife, Aetna, and Cigna, to name but a few, with these new plans setting up in-network providers agreeing to reduce their fees, and out-of-network providers accepting the new insurance benefits. Patients paid the difference between the provider's prices and the insurance payments.

PPO plans peaked in 2011 with a 65% market share but have been losing ground ever since. Presently, new insurance plans are offering lower and lower payouts, with the result that many dentists are dropping out of the networks, unable to run their businesses on these low payouts.

Patients need to know what insurance (if any) their dentist takes and choose carefully what plan, if any, they are going to sign up for. When it comes to deductibles, co-pays, and procedures not covered by insurance, many institutions in the US will provide financial help (loans) for what's not covered by insurance.

What are co-pays and deductibles? Do I really have to pay them?

Before your dental insurance starts paying, you must meet your deductible, the same as you must do with your medical insurance. Unlike medical insurance deductibles, which usually are several thousands of dollars, dental insurance co-pays are low—around $50 to $100.

After meeting your deductible, your dental insurance, depending on the plan you have purchased, can cover 50% to 100%, depending on the procedure.

Why do some dentists charge more than other dentists for the same procedure?

There is an iconic story of the artist Pablo Picasso sketching in a park. A bold woman approached the great man and said:

"It's you — Picasso, the great artist! Oh, you must sketch my portrait! I insist."

Picasso agreed to sketch her. After studying her for a moment, he used a single pencil stroke to create her portrait. He handed the woman his work of art.

"It's perfect!" she gushed. "You managed to capture my essence with one stroke, in one moment. Thank you! How much do I owe you?"

"Five thousand dollars," the artist replied.

"But, why?" the woman sputtered. "How could you want so much money for this picture? It only took you a second to draw it!"

To which Picasso responded: "Madame, it took me my entire life."

The experienced, skilled, and talented dentists usually charge higher fees. The location and cost of their office operation are also factors that determine their fees, but you are paying for the years these men and women spent studying and perfecting their skills, just like Picasso, to provide you with the best dental health . . . and a million-dollar smile.

Why should I see a dentist regularly? Do I really need a cleaning every six months?

Those dentist visits are preventive to keep your teeth and gums healthy. Cavities or tooth decay and periodontal disease—none of which you are able to see and not always able to feel in their early stages—are insidious and sometimes don't reveal their symptoms until you feel discomfort and pain . . . and by then you might be looking at complicated and costly procedures to address your dental health, such as a root canal or losing a tooth or teeth.

Also, your dentist can detect medical conditions if they see you on a regular basis. A dentist can recognize high blood pressure readings when taking a patient's blood pressure, malodor from diabetes, or a sore in the mouth that has not been healing that indicates leukemia.

CHAPTER 6

Dental Procedures

An initial comprehensive oral exam is conducted on new patients or every three years on existing patients. This exam is essential for the dentist so he or she can amass the necessary diagnostic tools they will need to determine an appropriate treatment plan for each individual's specific needs.

The exam consists of:

1. Completion of the medical and dental questionnaire and statement of chief complaint.
2. All recommended X-rays done by registered dental assistants or hygienist.
3. Review of medical and dental questionnaire and chief complaint by dentist.
4. Head and neck examination, looking for any abnormal lymph nodes, tender/sore spots. This is done by the dentist.
5. TMJ evaluation to look for any abnormal sounds such as clicking, popping, or rubbing bone on bone, pain, or soreness. Done by the dentist.

6.   Intraoral soft tissue examination of gingiva and mucosa, looking for any sign of infection and inflammation such as gingivitis and abscess. This is done by the dentist.

7.   Intraoral examination of hard tissues, including examination of teeth for any cavities; missing teeth; chipped and broken teeth; any signs of tooth wear because of grinding, bruxism, and clenching; any sign of infection in the bone around roots of the teeth; any impacted teeth; and bone loss from periodontal disease. All these procedures are done by the dentist.

8.   Oral cancer screening. Done by the dentist.

9.   Then the dentist reviews all the findings with the patient and formulates at least two treatment plans for the patient to choose from.

Beyond this, the dental procedures you might need could include:

Fillings or Dental Restorations – These are the most commonly used treatment modalities to treat dental caries or cavities. Tooth decay is the most prevalent chronic disease in adults. Cavities are caused by the bacteria in your mouth combining with the simple sugars from the foods you eat to create an acid that breaks down tooth enamel. Amalgam alloys, composite resin, porcelain, and gold are the most commonly used materials to fill or restore the teeth.

Cleaning – Just as you might perform a spring cleaning in your house, think of your dental cleaning as a regular cleaning of your teeth and gums. Generally, a dentist will recommend a regular cleaning for someone who does not have periodontal disease every six months. During these regular visits, most patients undergo a good regular cleaning, and for most of us, this surface cleaning is all one needs. The procedure usually focuses on eliminating bacteria, food particles, and tartar from the teeth and from those surfaces above the gum line. This type of cleaning is referred to as prophylaxis and is followed by a polishing of the teeth.

But there are levels a cleaning may take, beyond the usual one we have all had. Depending on the patient's immune system, type of bacteria, or microorganism living in the oral cavity—and their oral hygiene regimen—the patient might be suffering from periodontitis, which requires periodontal therapy or deep cleaning. This is a more complicated and involved procedure, but certainly necessary for teeth and gum health. Periodontitis, infection of the soft and hard tissue surrounding the tooth, if not treated, can lead to bone loss, loose teeth, and ultimately can end, if not treated, in tooth loss.

Periodontal disease is the leading cause of tooth loss.

Root Canals – Falling under the category of complex dental procedures, the purpose of a root canal is to save the tooth; it is the treatment of choice for teeth badly damaged either by trauma or tooth decay. In some cases, a toothache can also lead to a root canal treatment. Root canals or endodontic treatment involve removing the infected pulp tissue in the root of the tooth. Pulp tissue is a living tissue that consists of blood vessels, nerves (that's why teeth hurt), and lymphatic tissue. This procedure is usually a lengthy one and involves several small dental X-rays and more than one visit.

Bridges & Crowns – Bridges and crowns are nonremovable, what we call fixed prosthetics. Their function is exactly as their name implies:

a bridge spans (bridges) missing teeth spaces; a crown caps (crowns) a damaged or compromised tooth. A bridge is made up of two or more crowns that will attach to natural teeth sitting on either side of the space (these are called abutment teeth). The false teeth, or pontics, are made into that bridge, and the patient has the choice of what they want their crown or bridge to be made of (options range from porcelain, ceramic, or various metal alloys). The determination of what type of material used comes from where exactly the crown or bridge will go in your mouth, as well as the expense of the materials used.

Being fitted for both a bridge and a crown usually requires a two-visit dental procedure, the first being preparation and the making of an impression (mold). The impression is made for the dental lab so they can create the crown or bridge. During the second visit the dentist tries the crown or bridge in the patient's mouth, and if the fit is clinically accepted and the patient is happy with the way it looks and feels, then it is permanently cemented. Between the two visits, the patient will have a provisional or temporary. A temporary bridge or crown is constructed and fitted at that first visit to protect the area/tooth until the patient returns.

Implants – Think of the dental implants as posts. Throughout history, we have always been looking to somehow replace our missing teeth. As mentioned earlier, from finely shaped and polished wood to sea shells, all these materials and more were tried as early dental implants with no success. The modern-day titanium implants used since the 1970s have had unprecedented success. Today, ceramic implants are available depending on the case; ceramic is ideal for patients who object to having metals in their body, and in extremely rare cases, allergies. Implants are surgically placed in the edentulous area, with the number of implants varying from one to several, depending on the number of teeth missing, proposed treatment plan, and patient finances. Implants replace the root of the tooth and then receive a permanent crown, bridge, or denture. Implants can act just like natural teeth and can indeed support whatever replacement or bridge is fit onto them. Again, metals and ceramic materials are used in making implants, depending on where exactly in the mouth they are going. Patients usually tolerate the procedure well and have minimum pain post-surgery.

Dentures, Complete and Partial – From those old Poligrip commercials on TV and maybe from what adult patients have been exposed to from their own parents, we are pretty much all aware of dentures. We are also well aware of that sunken mouth look an older person can get when they no longer have any teeth in their mouth. Luckily, these days a person does not have to live with no teeth, few teeth, or old dentures that do not fit right.

There are basically three types of dentures (removable) used for specific purposes: a *full or complete* denture for patients who have no natural teeth remaining, a *partial* denture used to replace a few missing teeth, or an immediate denture or *temporary denture/transitional* dentures fitted immediately after a tooth or several teeth are extracted, used to replace these teeth as the mouth heals.

Complete dentures, immediate dentures, and transitional dentures are commonly made of an acrylic base and acrylic teeth. The color of denture base can be matched with the natural color of the gum and mucosa; for instance, darker-skin patients usually have darker-color soft tissues. The base of partial dentures are fabricated either from metal or acrylic, and teeth can be either acrylic or porcelain . . . with porcelain costing more.

Before a patient can be fitted for a partial denture, all other dental procedures they may need—cleaning, filling, being fitted for crowns—need to be completed. A patient's mouth must heal from these or any other dental procedures before the first impression (mold) is made of the mouth for the dentures.

TMD Treatment – Though we have all heard of the term TMJ, TMJ is not a malady. We all have TMJ, the three letters here representing the temporomandibular joint, which is a hinge that connects our lower jaw (mandible) to the temporal bones of the skull, right in front of each ear. If you place your fingers gently on either side of your head, just in front of your ears, and then open and close your mouth, you should be able to feel a joint moving. This is your temporomandibular joint, or TMJ. TMD or temporomandibular disorders are really what people mean when they complain about TMJ. Unfortunately, these joints have a habit of causing problems in humans, particularly as these joints are never really still, even when we sleep. TMJ disorders can be painful and can include strange symptoms such as headaches and ear pain, as well as the more common sounds of clicking, popping, or grating. These symptoms can be on one side or both sides of the face and can occur when chewing, opening or closing the mouth, or even when someone is at rest.

Review of a patient's medical and dental history, physical exam, X-ray, CAT Scan, MRI, etc. can be helpful in arriving at a diagnosis of TMJ conditions.

If you have ever suffered from jaw pain, you know it is not pleasant, which is why it is important that you make an appointment with a dentist if you suspect you may suffer from a TMJ disorder. Although occasionally these disorders will go away by themselves, more commonly the patient who suffers from TMJ disorder requires some treatment. Your dentist may recommend gentle treatments at the outset, such as resting the jaw and avoiding hard and crunchy foods. Stress management, jaw exercises, and other techniques such as massage also may be prescribed to help the patient deal with the problem. Treatment also can consist of the correction of the bite either by orthodontic or restorative treatment, custom-made splints such as a night guard, anti-inflammatory agents, or a combination of all of these. Not all TMD can be treated by routine dental care, though usually your dentist will finish the evaluation and refer you to a specialist appropriate if you do indeed exhibit symptoms of TMD he or she cannot treat.

Trauma, habits such as grinding and clenching, derangement of the disk and skeletal components, stress, and arthritis are some of the causes of this disorder.

Please don't wait until this problem gets any worse if you already suffer from pain in your jaw. A quick visit to the orthodontist could help you solve the problem, removing this pain from your life altogether.

Extractions – Simply put, an extraction is a dental procedure that involves the removal or pulling of a tooth. Dental extractions are performed for several reasons: either the tooth structure or the periodontal structure (the bone and gum that hold the tooth) is severely damaged, the position of the tooth might be impacted, or as is true in some cases, a patient might not be able to afford a more complex treatment such as a root canal to save the tooth. Any dentist's primary objective is to do whatever he or she can to save a tooth. But if a patient has a broken a tooth that can't be capped, an infection has worked its way in too deeply into the gum and root, wisdom teeth are impacted and causing pain (as they so often do in adults), or if the patient is suffering from an abscess, a tooth might well need to be pulled.

CHAPTER 7

Improve Your Appearance, Improve Your Life

Any good dentist is interested in saving all of your natural teeth. But natural teeth aren't always attractive teeth. They can be individually crooked, out of alignment with each other, have gaps between them, and be discolored. That's where orthodontics (braces) and cosmetic dentistry can help you get the smile of your dreams.

Orthodontics and the Adult Patient

What is Orthodontics?

Orthodontics is a specific discipline of dentistry that deals with diagnosing and treating the irregularities of the teeth and the alignment of the jaw. It is also the one discipline of dentistry that adult patients often overlook beyond all others. Getting a cavity filled, maybe even stopping in for a quick six-month visit is one thing, but many adults simply do not think straightening their teeth is something they need to do. As it is, so many adults avoid the dentist, and it's easy to understand why. In the past, some methods of correcting teeth were painful, making going to the dentist something to avoid and certainly not something to enjoy. Even our favorite movies seem to enjoy making dentistry into some horror-filled experience that should be avoided at all costs. It's no wonder adults who haven't been to a dentist in a good long while, who already fear the dentist, would want to avoid seeing an orthodontist for what they view as extra dental treatment.

The good news for you today is that dentistry has changed and orthodontic treatments specifically are no longer the long, painful processes they once were. The adult patient doesn't have to view teeth straightening as something extra to simple dental care. The new technologies we offer today mean that your teeth can be gently corrected using an assortment of different strategies, with little to no pain or discomfort. And the aesthetics of orthodontic procedures have evolved so much that the adult patient need not concern themselves any longer about having to endure the classic mouthful of metal.

Here are just ten benefits a patient can enjoy from modern orthodontics:

1. **A dream smile**. Can you imagine waking up in the morning, looking in the mirror to see the smile you have always dreamed of looking right back at you? With today's modern tools and techniques, we can correct almost every problem with misaligned teeth to give you a smile to be proud of.

2. **Improved self-confidence**. There's nothing like a beautiful smile to make you feel gorgeous and more confident in yourself; this is true whether you are an adult or a child. Both adults and children alike benefit from the improved sense of self-worth of corrective orthodontic work.

3. **Better functionality**. A corrected bite can make it easier to enjoy the foods you love by making your teeth more usable in your day-to-day life.

4. **Reduced muscle and jaw strain**. Jaw ache is truly unpleasant pain, one that seems to take over your whole face and leave you uncomfortable for hours. A tooth correction now could reduce the strain on your jaw and the muscles surrounding it, eliminating this sort of pain for good.

5. **Less risk of future problems**. Taking the time to correct your teeth now could help prevent a multitude of future issues, from jaw surgery to premature tooth loss.

6. **Increased ability to keep teeth clean**. Keeping your teeth clean is vitally important to reduce the risk of tooth decay and gum disease, which in turn can lead to more serious conditions. With teeth that are crowded or too spaced out, keeping them as clean as they should be can be difficult.

7. **Long-term healthiness in your mouth**. Correcting misaligned teeth will help to keep your mouth healthy; you'll be able to keep your teeth cleaner, and the closing of gaps will stop dangerous bacteria from building up around your gums. This can also help to prevent you from contracting a gum disease that could, in turn, lead to far more serious health conditions. Increased ability to keep your teeth clean combined with the correct positioning of teeth within your mouth will lead to better long-term dental health.

8. **Reduced risk of future tooth extraction**. No one likes having a tooth pulled. Even with painkillers, it can still be a painful and

distressing experience. Having your teeth corrected with orthodontic techniques early will drastically reduce, or even eliminate, the need to have teeth pulled in the future.

9. **Look younger longer.** Our teeth help to support our facial structure. If they fall out, your mouth can sink in, and your cheeks sag from lack of support. This can make you look older than your years. Failing to correct the problems that you have with your teeth now could lead to this premature loss of teeth, and therefore the appearance of aging before your time.

10. **Improved quality of life.** Having straight and healthy teeth gives you more confidence and higher self-esteem to help advance your career path and build relationships with others. Straight teeth are also easier to keep clean to avoid dental problems in the future.

What's holding adult patients from reaping these benefits today?

"I can't afford orthodontic treatments."

"I don't want to wear braces."

"I don't have the time for a long course of treatment."

"I'm scared of the dentist."

"My teeth aren't that bad."

These are all reasons to avoid the dentist or orthodontist that we have heard time and time again. And they are all reasons your dentist can help you overcome with his or her knowledge, skill, and confidence that a better smile awaits you.

CHAPTER 8

Q&A:
Orthodontic Basics

What causes crooked or spaced teeth?

The causes of crooked teeth vary from person to person. Many conditions are inherited from our parents, such as missing teeth, impacted teeth, teeth crowding, mismatched tooth size and jaw size, spacing and protrusion of teeth and jaws; there's not much anyone can do to prevent these hereditary issues, though they can certainly be corrected.

In other cases, the causes of crooked teeth can stem from habits that you may have had as a young child, such as thumb or pacifier sucking.

Another cause of misaligned smiles can be a patient losing their baby teeth before their adult teeth were ready to erupt.

Losing a permanent tooth often causes the neighboring and opposing teeth to drift to occupy the space, causing misalignment of teeth.

Periodontal disease often results in bone loss in the jaw; teeth then drift to abnormal positions.

Some of these problems can crop up at any stage of your life, causing your smile to degenerate and prompting that all-important first visit to

the dentist. It doesn't matter where the problem came from; in orthodontic procedures you will read about below, you can still get the smile
of your dreams.

Do crooked teeth cause cavities or gum problems?

Crooked and misaligned teeth are not just an aesthetic concern; they
can also contribute to dental and gum problems. Crooked teeth do not
cause cavities and gum disease by themselves, but . . . as with all dental
problems, crooked teeth can contribute to a slippery slope of complications. At the basic end, overcrowding and misaligned teeth can cause
significant difficulty for the person trying to clean their teeth properly.
Toothbrushes and floss are extremely hard to manipulate around a
mouth full of nooks and crannies that are overcrowded or misaligned.
An improper at-home teeth cleaning regimen, even if done regularly,
can all too easily lead to bacteria growth. This bacteria, if not treated,
can grow into gingivitis or periodontal disease and tooth decay. If gums
don't fit securely around teeth, there is more space for that bacteria to
grow. The difficulty with brushing and flossing becomes much more
problematic for adult patients with medical problems such as arthritis,
Parkinson's disease, multiple sclerosis, or carpal tunnel syndrome.

When should I have an orthodontic evaluation?

The American Dental Association recommends that children should
have an orthodontic evaluation by the age of seven. Getting kids into
the dentist at this age allows the dentist to spot any problems that may
develop as the adult teeth take their place. Does that mean it is too late
for adults to have braces? Absolutely not. As an adult, you too could

enjoy the treatments that can restore your smile to full health. It's equally important for you to make an appointment as soon as possible to prevent your teeth from degenerating further.

I always wanted to have straight shining teeth; my parents could not afford braces, and I got married and had children. As a parent they came first. My husband and I took care of them, and now they are all grown up, have college degrees, and are working. Now it's our turn. Can we still have straight teeth?

The short answer here is: yes. No matter how old you are, overall dental health and the aesthetics of your smile can be improved. As long as an adult has good, healthy teeth and equally healthy supporting structure (bone and soft tissue, gingiva or gum) they can undergo orthodontic treatment and be fitted for braces. Today there are various types of orthodontic appliances in addition to metal braces available that can satisfy the needs of adult patients during treatment. Ceramic braces, lingual braces, and Invisalign are most commonly used in adult patients with equal success to traditional metal or silver braces.

Aren't braces expensive?

They may seem to be expensive at first, but they are worth it; braces are an investment that can last a lifetime. The long-term benefits such as increased self-confidence that we gain from beautiful, straight teeth, better bite, better chewing, and even clearer speaking outweigh the cost. Patients that are interested in the benefits of straight teeth should think of getting braces as an investment in *themselves*. In some cases, orthodontic treatment can save tooth structure, avoid additional dental procedures, and save money and time in both the short and long term.

After my braces are removed, will my teeth stay in the newly aligned, perfect position forever?

Our teeth are always moving. For many patients, retainers are prescribed for future use to help maintain the good work your braces did.

What are retainers?

Teeth are stubborn. As mentioned above, they always move. After orthodontic treatment is completed, to prevent movement, patients are fitted with a device called a retainer. There are several types of retainers available: fixed retainers, Hawley retainers, and clear Essix retainers (similar to Invisalign aligners) are the most widely used.

Is it true that the tighter you set my braces, the faster they work and the sooner I can get them off?

Braces that are too tight are not good for your teeth, and a tighter fit doesn't mean you will be adjusted any faster. Braces are tightened to the tension that will work best for each patient's need, and at the same time be the most comfortable.

Couldn't my family DDS perform all of these orthodontic procedures?

Yes, he or she might be familiar with orthodontic treatment. Remember the dentist works for you. Patients can and should find out about their dentists' experience in orthodontics. Ask if they have done similar cases to yours and if they have before and after picture/records. You want to seek out the professional who has had years of schooling in this area, who knows these procedures like the back of his or her hand, and who performs them on a daily basis. Some of what you read of the procedures that follow are very complex. You want the person attending to your orthodontic dental care to be knowledgeable and experienced in what they do, don't you?

CHAPTER 9

Types of Braces

Taking into account the "I'm too old for braces" myth, one of the biggest concerns adult patients have in considering braces is how they might look after they get their braces on. Luckily, there have been some amazing advances in braces technology, and as I have seen time and again, when the adult patient learns about all the options presently available, they are usually quite open to (and most importantly will open their mouth to) being fitted for braces, knowing the result will be something quite fantastic.

Traditional/Metal braces. That mouthful of metal; large, dark silver brackets or rings around teeth, around the front teeth especially, and clunky wires that adults remember with horror have been replaced with modern small and less noticeable smart brackets which are made of either highly polished stainless steel or clear materials. These smart brackets are specifically designed to guide the teeth gently to a proper position which they should naturally fall into by themselves. Modern arch wires (the actual source of the force that moves teeth) are made of nickel titanium, stainless steel, or titanium alloy that move teeth faster and easier with no or minimum discomfort to patients. They also shorten treatment duration substantially compared to braces and wires of the past. These are still the most commonly used type of braces.

Clear braces are cosmetically pleasing and less visible. They work almost as efficiently as stainless steel braces. Though pretty much the same size and shape of traditional braces, the brackets here can be either tooth enamel white or clear so as to blend in better with the patient's teeth. We can even use enamel-colored wire for even better blending. Clear braces are either plastic or ceramic. Ceramic braces are more expensive and because of their abrasive nature are not generally recommend for use on lower teeth. Ceramic brackets on lower teeth can abrade upper teeth and cause irreversible damage to the enamel. Clear plastic braces usually stain. For the adult patient who smokes or drinks coffee, red wine, or colored beverages, this usually poses a concern. Make sure to ask your dentist if the clear braces that he/she uses stain or not.

Lingual braces are another option for adults with high aesthetic demands. Envision traditional braces but placed on the inside of the teeth. Lingual braces are recommended to patients who tend toward diligent teeth cleaning, as braces on the inside of the teeth are harder to clean. Lingual braces can be more uncomfortable at first; adjustments take more time, treatment duration is longer, and they are a more costly investment. But lingual braces are great for adults worried about the look of braces in their mouths, as these kinds of braces are virtually hidden.

Invisalign look very much like clear mouth guards (plastic trays called aligners) and are more comfortable than any of the braces discussed above. Fitted with an average of twenty or so aligners (the number of Invisalign is determined by the severity of the case), dental hygiene regimens are easier with these braces since they can be removed when one brushes and flosses. Replaced usually at bimonthly intervals, the patient wearing Invisalign interacts with their dentist on a more regular basis when wearing this kind of braces. The downside here is that Invisaligns will not work on more acute dental concerns, and they are more expensive than other braces except lingual braces. Treatment duration with Invisalign is usually longer, and the patient may require braces to finish the treatment. The technology of Invisalign is advancing rapidly, and in the author's opinion, it will be the treatment of choice for almost any case in the near future.

For braces that are nearly undetectable—for all intents and purposes invisible—Invisalign is the best option.

CHAPTER 10

Cosmetic Procedures

All dental care has a cosmetic component to it. Anyone who works on your teeth, from the dental hygienist who cleans them to the orthodontist who straightens them, is working hard to make sure your mouth functions properly, that you can enjoy the full and comfortable range of your bite, and that you will be free of gum disease. But these dental pros also want you to be able to flash your beautiful white smile as much as you can.

Given the above, there are dental procedures that are purely cosmetic in nature. Some adults are lucky enough to come to a dentist needing no real treatment, cavity filling, root canal work, just simple check-ups and cleaning , only seeing a dentist for a cosmetic concern.

The thing to remember about the procedures that follow is that like orthodontics, almost anyone at any age can benefit from cosmetic dentistry. The dental procedures falling only under the cosmetic umbrella are:

Teeth Whitening

Surely there are kits available at any pharmacy for anyone who wishes to whiten their teeth at home, but when visiting a dentist for professional teeth whitening (what we call chairside bleaching), the patient submits to a teeth whitening procedure they simply can't get over the counter. Having a dentist perform teeth whitening, you can be assured that not only do you have skilled hands in your mouth, but you'll also enjoy the added benefit of having a doctor apply and examine the whitening process from angles you'd simply never be able to see.

There are a whole host of factors that work at dulling or staining the enamel of our teeth; the older we get, the more the enamel of our teeth can fade. Smoking, alcohol and coffee drinking, diet and poor health, and medications can stain teeth and lead to discoloration; some people are prone to a lightening of the white of their enamel over time. Yes, sometimes a deeper, more serious dental issue can lead to tooth discolorations—abscesses or overall tooth decay to name two—and chairside bleaching would merely mask those problems. But if you are someone with a healthy mouth whose teeth happen to be dulling, chairside bleaching can make a vast improvement in your smile.

As with all procedures, we conduct an initial dental exam, taking digital X-rays to determine what exactly is causing your discoloration. Barring any serious issue as mentioned above, we proceed with the whitening process to lighten your teeth to the most natural white shade that fits the whites of your eyes.

It's almost a painless procedure where a protective material—usually a gel or a rubber shield—is put across the soft tissue of your mouth (lips and gums) while the dentist keeps your teeth exposed. A bleaching agent is then applied to the teeth with a special light used to enhance the action of that agent.

For the desired effect, chairside bleaching might take more than one dental visit and more than one hour a time.

Q&A: Bleaching

How long will the bleaching last?

No bleaching lasts forever, and generally, the longevity of the whitening is once again aided by your oral hygiene regimen.

Is a patient's age a factor in bleaching?

Again, allowing for generally healthy teeth and gums, patients older than age sixteen can benefit from teeth whitening. (Whitening is not recommended for patients younger than sixteen.) True, an older patient may have had more time to stain his or her teeth by coffee drinking, smoking, and maybe bad general health.

I only have one or two teeth that are dark; how do we whiten them?

Single teeth that appear dark often indicate some disease attacking that tooth. If the tooth is dead (for instance the tooth needs a root canal), it can be whitened from the inside. If the tooth is still alive, you don't need a root canal for it, and single-tooth bleaching would be recommended in this case. Matching the whiteness of the surrounding teeth is a trickier process, though.

My crowns/the teeth in my bridge are stained as well. Can teeth bleaching make them whiter?

Whitening agents only work on your natural teeth. Resins or any other materials used as restoration material cannot be whitened with teeth bleaching agents.

CHAPTER 11

Porcelain Veneers

As popular as Invisalign are in modern orthodontics, veneers are right up there on the list of popular cosmetic dental applications. A popular choice for most of the celebrities you see beaming their perfect smiles at you from your television, these thin shells of enamel-colored ceramic coverings have become the go-to for many everyday guy or gal looking to present the perfect modern smile. Bonding to the front of the teeth, veneers address the full aesthetic of your mouth. Veneers can be used to cover, reshape, or cosmetically enhance:

- gaps or spaces
- stains or discoloration
- chips, cracks, pits, and even fractures
- crooked or otherwise poorly positioned teeth

Veneers also can be used as a substitute for orthodontic braces.

Adults with small gaps and minor alignment issues who prefer to avoid the time and appearance of braces now have an option that can change the size and shape of their teeth. Some dentists call veneers "instant orthodontics" because you can have an immediate correction of crooked or crowded front teeth. They can alter the shape of your face and the appearance of your smile by adjusting the size of your teeth.

Types of veneers include:

- *Porcelain veneers* – allowing the dentist to give you the smile of your dreams by changing the shape, crookedness, color, and spacing of your teeth in just two visits;
- *Lumineers* – these veneers are super thin yet ultra-strong porcelain veneers that change your smile from dull to dazzling in the most comfortable way possible. In many instances, no shots are required. Lumineers veneers in selective cases don't require much smoothing of your tooth, so they don't compromise the tooth structure itself.

The benefits of veneers are many. They will not stain, are durable, last many years, are strong enough so you can chew food just as you would with your natural teeth, look just like natural teeth, and provide an immediate solution to teeth whitening.

To be sure, veneers are on the higher end of the price scale when it comes to overall modern dental procedures.

Years ago, when a patient wanted cosmetic correction of crowded or poorly shaped teeth, he or she often had crowns placed to recontour (reshape) them. However, this involves removing a lot of the solid good tooth structure just for cosmetic reasons. Veneers can be placed with either little or no removal of enamel; the procedure is very conservative.

Q&A: Veneers

How do I know how many veneers I need?

The number of veneers a patient gets is entirely dependent on the patient. They can use only one for a chipped, discolored tooth or as many teeth as patients desire. Usually, dentists recommend placing veneers on all visible teeth when the patient smiles to have a harmonious smile. It can be four to six front teeth and then as many of the back teeth that are visible in a natural smile.

How long will my veneers last?

Veneers are durable and last a long time; they are made of tough stuff indeed. And of course, once again, if you are proactive in your dental care, they can last a long time.

I got my veneers because my teeth were chipped and stained; can veneers chip and stain?

Porcelain veneers should not stain, but though the porcelain is a strong substance, it is a form of glass and like glass can chip if you don't take proper care in biting down on hard foods.

CHAPTER 12

Composite or Teeth Bonding

Composite bonding is the process of adhering a tooth-colored resin by a high-intensity curing light. Typically used cosmetically to improve the appearance or shape of one tooth, the resin attached will as much improve how a tooth looks as add to its overall strength. Decidedly cheaper than veneers and addressing one or more teeth, we also use teeth bonding to close gaps between teeth. The disadvantage of the composite bonding includes discoloration that can come from a patient's dental regimen, smoking, or diet. Also, the results are highly dependent on the clinical and technical skills of the dentist.

Q&A: Bonding

How long does bonding last?

Though made of a sturdy material and a less expensive cosmetic fix than other procedures, bonding does not last as long as crowns and veneers.

Behzad Nazari, DDS

Can any tooth be bonded?

As a general answer, yes, but the best teeth for this process are ones where you exert the lowest degree of pressure when chewing. Therefore bonding tends to work better on front teeth than back teeth.

CHAPTER 13

Veneers, Bonding, or Braces: Which Is Right for Me?

In cases of patients with more severe alignment issues, braces or Invisalign are the treatment of choice. In these type of cases, teeth structures are saved since to bring them into alignment without orthodontic treatment, the dentist has to prepare (reshape) the teeth more than usual, which may lead to teeth sensitivity, root canals, and crowns. At the same time, if the teeth are chipped, discolored, or the patient is not happy with the shape of their teeth, orthodontics, veneers, or bonding is necessary.

The patient who presents with minor gaps and alignment issues can receive either veneers, bonding, or braces.

As mentioned before, if the teeth are discolored, chipped, or the patient does not like the shape of the teeth but doesn't have alignment issues, veneers or bonding are the treatment of choice.

CHAPTER 14

Overcoming Your Fear of the Dentist

By now you should realize that your dentist is here to help you and your entire family with custom treatments specifically designed to give you back your smile. But if you still struggle with an overwhelming fear of the dentist, then even the thought of taking that first step into the office could be difficult for you.

Here are some methods to help allay your fears of seeing a dentist.

1. Ask Questions. The most common reason for fear is a simple lack of understanding. If your only knowledge of braces comes from a person who had them fitted twenty years ago when technology was far less advanced, then you will understandably be concerned. You can ask questions of your orthodontist in an initial consultation or even over the phone. They will explain exactly what a procedure entails.

2. Do Your Research. If your fear of the dentist borders on the level of a phobia, then it is worth researching local orthodontists in your area that are especially used to coping with nervous patients. You also

may be able to take advantage of a method of sedation or discover more information about the best pain relief to prevent you from feeling anything during your procedure.

3. Take the First Step. Your fear could be the one thing holding you back from the smile you have always dreamed of and longed for. Don't let fear hold you back from great dental health. Make that first appointment and explain to your doctor how you feel. You can be sure that you will be made to feel completely comfortable and at ease.

4. Your dentist is there to help you, not to harm you. You may have been putting off this your dental visit for years. Now is the time to take your first step to correcting your dental issues and putting your life back on track.

CHAPTER 15

Case Studies

The purpose of including the three case studies below is to illustrate the fact no one is too old for a million-dollar smile. Though the cases below are not discussed in a typical manner that one may find in a scientific journal or textbook, the medical history of every single patient has been thoroughly reviewed and when necessary appropriate medical clearances were obtained. All necessary dental records such as X-rays, detailed pictures, study models, and periodontal assessment were gathered to best determine what different treatment options were available; these were then discussed with the patients. In many cases, you will see that treatment followed over a longer period than just one or two visits.

Most of these patients presented to our clinic for a specific complaint/ problem. They were not seeking a complete smile makeover, but after a thorough evaluation of their dental needs and informing the patient what modern-day dentistry could offer them, they decided to seek and subsequently came to enjoy their million-dollar smile. You will also see that in all three cases, as with so many patients who present to our office, time and again the results were better than the patient ever could have dreamed.

All of the restorative (treating cavities with fillings, etc.) and gum treatment were completed before any cosmetic or orthodontic treatment ensued. The treatment plans presented below are the ones the patient chose from the treatment options we offered.

Following are a few of the real-life cases we have seen:

1. An eighty-two-year-old Hispanic woman presented with her chief complaint, a pain in her upper left canine area, thinking that her upper partial denture needed adjustment. A full-mouth X-ray series was obtained and a clinical exam performed, but a review of this patient's medical history revealed that she had been on several medications to control her high blood pressure, heart rate, diabetes mellitus, arthritis, and high cholesterol. These medications are well known to cause dry mouth, a fact needing to be addressed. Regardless of the type of dental treatment, saliva substitutes and a suggestion for the patient to drink plenty of water was prescribed.

    On clinical exam and review of X-rays, it was discovered that the patient had cervical caries (a particular type of tooth decay that attacks bone tissue) of tooth number # 11, which explained the pain. Cervical caries is a typical finding in elderly patients, which must be addressed both by physicians prescribing medications and general dentists, once again affirming the fact that dentists caring for this specific age population must have a good grasp of pharmacology, dental implications of medications, and disease processes. The endodontic treatment for tooth #11 was prescribed, and upon patient acceptance of treatment and obtaining a medical release from her primary care physician, this treatment was performed successfully.

After completion of the endodontic treatment—which eliminated her pain—the patient complained of her lower denture: "It does not fit good and I cannot chew good with this." After an evaluation of her partial, implants were recommended, though the patient had been convinced she would not be eligible for an implant because of her advanced age. The patient was surprised and happy to learn otherwise and received two implants and a lower complete denture.

2. A sixty-three-year-old Caucasian female came to our office for a routine dental exam and cleaning. The patient presented with adult localized moderate periodontal disease, several inter proximal caries, and missing teeth, which she wanted to replace. She also presented with severely crowded upper and lower teeth. Added to the above, arthritis in this woman's hands made it hard for her to floss properly.

Upon a thorough examination, we presented several treatment options, with the ideal option a two-phase treatment plan.

The first stage would be to complete the periodontal and restorative treatment, and the second to have the lady receive orthodontic treatment to relieve and correct her crowding issues. With the crowding eliminated it would be much easier for her to brush and floss, in turn helping to control her periodontal disease.

During the interview the patient stated that she had always wanted to have straight teeth, but something had always prevented her from getting braces: helping her husband with mortgage payments, going back to school to get her real estate license, taking care of her kids, and later their college and divorces. Like many adults, this patient did so want a great big gorgeous smile but simply figured she was too old for it and that older patients couldn't have braces. After showing her many adult patients who had received orthodontic treatment and had life-changing outcomes, the patient was interested in entertaining the idea of braces after we completed the periodontal and restorative treatment.

In the two years of completion of her treatment, this patient has been extremely satisfied with her decision to undergo all the procedures we have managed for her—battling her periodontal disease, replacing and fixing her teeth, alleviating her overcrowding through braces and other orthodontic procedures, fitting her for implants—and now smiles all the time.

3. A male Hispanic patient presented for consultation, hoping to have his removable partial dentures adjusted. He showed up with a bag full of partials that he had received from several dental offices, none of which he had ever been happy with for a multitude of reasons. A clinical exam and X-ray revealed that the teeth adjacent to the areas where the denture fitting had drifted, and placing a partial that could be put in and removed comfortably was near to impossible. Uprighting and aligning the teeth with braces (orthodontic treatment) was discussed with the patient, but as so many adults before him, he did not believe he could get braces; he was more embarrassed over the idea than anything else. After discussing what

braces could do for his teeth (uprighting and aligning the posterior teeth, relieving the crowding in the front teeth) and him seeing other older patients with braces, the patient agreed to discuss with his wife the procedures we were suggesting. A few days later this patient began orthodontic treatment, and after almost twenty-two months of orthodontic treatment, he received new partials that fit better and were easier to insert and remove, as he had much less space between the partial and his teeth after we were done. Less food was being trapped in his gums as well.

Again, here was another adult patient who never thought he would wear braces.

Conclusion

Every tooth in a man's head is more valuable than a diamond.
~Miguel de Cervantes

Are you smiling after reading this book? Do you feel now that there are possibilities for your dental health that you never considered before? Are you looking in the mirror right now trying to imagine what you would look like with that million-dollar smile?

Well, if you have learned anything from what you have just read, you don't have to just imagine it any longer! Lots of terminology and concepts were thrown at you in the preceding pages, but if you come away with one thing, it should be that you can indeed have that smile you have always wanted or that you thought was long gone from your life.

And your dentist can get it for you.

Dentistry has been around since the beginning of civilization, and we have seen that human beings have always been intrigued by the power of the smile. Even centuries ago, men and women were making changes to their teeth to get attention, to increase the beauty and "wattage" of their smile, and to stand out in the crowd with the beauty of their teeth. Celebrities sporting rows of Invisalign or the makers of teeth-whitening products might think they are riding the wave of something new, but as we have seen, cosmetic dentistry is not something new.

Simply put, for as long as humankind has had the ability to smile, which we seem to have always had, we have been interested in showing it off.

As adults, we have a unique perspective on life, gained from what we have gone through as much as what we can imagine might be coming. As children, we tend to see the world mainly as what is happening presently, but as adults we hopefully learn from the past and see a clearer route to the future. Of course, as adults, we have built up years of assumptions and tend to dig in our heels to what we want to believe, even if it's not true or doesn't serve us best in the long run.

We hope this book has helped you see where some of your assumptions and fears might not be warranted when getting back to the dentist or making dental visits should be a more regular part of your life.

There is nothing to hold you back now from that million-dollar smile.

Highly dedicated dental healthcare professionals specializing in adult care are out there, ready to take that journey with you, be it for a few visits or for a comprehensive treatment that might take a bit more time. From the simplest of dental procedures—like coming in for a check-up and regular cleaning—to being fitted for veneers or an implant, to finally getting braces—even at the ripe old age of fifty!—no matter what you need, as you have seen, it is all possible with modern dentistry.

A dentist enjoys a true one-of-a-kind perspective . . . his or her good work is as plain as the smile on their patient's face. You can surely benefit from the result of this noble work. Soon all you'll have to do is look in the mirror and see that no, you were not too old for that **MILLION-DOLLAR SMILE.**

Glossary of Dental Terms

abutment: A support for a dental prosthesis; typically, a tooth or implant is utilized as a fixture or *abutment* to secure that prosthesis to a specific place in the patient's mouth.

ADA: The abbreviation for the *American Dental Association.*

adjunctive: Any secondary treatment to the primary treatment a dentist performs.

administrative costs: These costs refer to *in-office* expenses and are unrelated to dental procedures and/or treatments provided by a dentist or dental associate.

amalgam: The hard alloy dentists often use to fill cavities. Amalgam is usually made of mercury, silver, tin or copper, and mixed with other metallic elements.

anesthesia: Drugs used to induce a state of near or complete unconsciousness.

bleaching: A dental process used to restore the white color of a patient's teeth, or to lighten stains or other discolorations that may have occurred with age or abuse. Bleaching is used in short and long-term applications or even through over-the-counter methods the layperson can employ.

bonding: A dental procedure where two (or more components) are integrated into a patient's mouth through mechanical and/or chemical means.

calculus: Also called *tartar,* these deposits attach to teeth as well as dental prosthetics; it is formed from minerals secreted by saliva.

cavity: Basically a *hole in a tooth*, caused by various forms of tooth erosion and decay.

composite: Any man-made material a dentist uses that is made up of more than one kind of substance.

co-payment: The patient's remaining balance of a dentist's bill after his or her insurance has paid its portion of that bill.

cosmetic dentistry: Dental procedures serving to only improve the appearance of a patient's mouth.

crown: A dental prosthesis is used to restore a tooth structure or to cover an implant; cemented into the patient's mouth or secured by some mechanical procedure, it is typically made of metal or ceramic, or combination of these materials.

decay: The decomposition of a tooth structure.

dental insurance: A health plan to assist a patient in paying the costs of dental procedures.

denture: A lab-made prosthesis, either secured permanently in a patient's mouth or created for temporary use and implantation replacing natural teeth and gum tissue.

enamel: This hardest substance of the human body is one of four components that make up teeth, the three others being dentin, cementum, and dental pulp.

endodontics: The dental specialty dealing with the study of and procedures used to treat the pulp or soft inner tissue of teeth.

endodontist: A dentist who specializes in endodontics.

filling: A lay term used for the materials (metal, alloy, plastic, or porcelain) used by a dentist to *fill* a cavity.

gingiva: Also known as the *gum*, this soft tissue of the mouth covers the border of the jaw that bears the patient's teeth.

gingivectomy: The dental procedure for removing or decreasing gingiva.

gingivitis: A disease where the patient's gum is inflamed but has not lost connective tissue.

impacted tooth: A tooth that is positioned in such a way that is *stuck* against another tooth, bone, or gum.

implant: A support, placed in the jaw, to hold a crown, bridge or denture.

inlay: Placed in the center of the tooth, gold, composite or porcelain is used to repair teeth damaged beyond being able to be fixed by a filling, but not needing a crown.

malocclusion: When the biting or chewing surfaces of upper and lower teeth are misaligned.

molar: The back teeth of the mouth used for grinding food.

occlusion: The contact that occurs in the biting (and chewing) of the upper and lower teeth.

onlay: Gold, composite or porcelain used to repair the outside areas of a tooth.

orthodontist: A dentist specializing in treating the misalignment of the mouth.

palate: The soft tissue roof of the mouth.

periodontal disease: Inflammatory gum disease (gingivitis) that has spread to the patient's bone.

periodontist: A dental specialist treating periodontal disease and other concerns of the gum and teeth.

plaque: Made (mostly) of bacteria, this colorless 'film' forms on teeth when a patient ingests too many foods high in sugars and starches and does not keep to a regular brushing regiment.

pontic: The artificial tooth on a permanent partial denture.

post: A rod inserted into an affected tooth's root to which a dentist can attach a various number of prosthesis or even a filling to restore the tooth structure.

preventive dentistry: Dental procedures that promote oral health and stave off or completely eliminate diseases incurred by patients in the normal passage of their lifetime.

pulp: Tissue in teeth that contain blood vessels and nerves.

resin, acrylic: Material used in various dental restorations and other procedures.

root canal: A procedure used when a tooth is decayed beyond the point of filling or fixing. In this two-step procedure a dentist removes the pulp of the tooth and then cleans and seals the inside of the tooth.

scaling: The process where a dentist uses certain instruments and even machines to remove plaque, calculus, and stains from a patient's teeth.

temporary removable denture: A prosthesis designed for temporary use.

temporomandibular: The connecting jaw joint that stretches from the base of the skull to the lower jaw.

temporomandibular joint dysfunction: Often called TMJ, which only refers to the actual temporomandibular joint, this is the malady occurring from a nonfunctioning temporomandibular joint.

unerupted: Generally called *impacted*, these are teeth that have formed but have not *surfaced* into the mouth.

uprighting: An orthodontic procedure used to make a tooth straighter.

About the Author

Behzad Nazari, DDS, is a dentist with eighteen years of experience serving Houston-area patients. He began his career as a registered pharmacist (RPh) after graduating from Texas Southern University in 1991. He then decided to pursue dentistry, eventually graduating with honors and a Doctor of Dental Surgery (DDS) from the University of Texas at Houston Dental Branch in 1998. In 2000, Dr. Nazari envisioned an all-in-one dental health center that could serve patients of all ages with a variety of dental and orthodontic services. That is when he founded Antoine Dental Center, which has since served thousands of patients in the greater Houston area.

Dr. Nazari teaches that comprehensive preventive care is one of the most important keys to good oral health. He believes it is never too late for a healthy, beautiful smile. His dedication to excellent care has led him to complete more than 1,800 hours of continuing education, with more than five hundred hours in orthodontics, occlusion, and TMJ correction alone. He is a proud member of the American Dental Association, the Texas Dental Association, the Greater Houston Dental Society, and the Academy of General Dentistry. He has completed several continuing education courses in orthodontics, implant dentistry, and cosmetic dentistry, and he is a graduate of the prestigious Kois Center training facility in Seattle, Washington.

Appendix

These patients, ranging in age from 42 to 82, came to our clinic for a specific complaint; they were not seeking a complete smile 'make over.'

It was only after a thorough evaluation of their dental needs, when they were assured that their initial concerns would be dealt with and that they would enjoy the further benefits of a Million Dollar Smile that we went ahead to completely restore their confidence, smile and outlook on life.

All of the restorative procedures they needed-treating filling cavities, gum treatment, etc., were completed before any cosmetic or orthodontic treatment ensued.

Case 1, 2 and 3: Restorative and gum treatment was followed by orthodontic treatment, cosmetic treatment being last.

Case 1

BEFORE	AFTER

Case 2

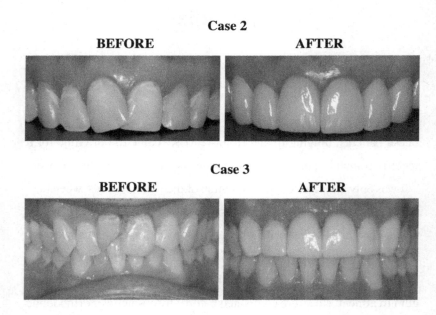

Case 4: Restorative and gum treatment was followed by orthodontic treatment. We found the patient thrilled with the outcome, especially seeing as no further treatment, such as bleaching or veneers was need.

Case 4: Restorative and gum treatment was followed by orthodontic treatment. We found the patient thrilled with the outcome, especially seeing as no further treatment, such as bleaching or veneers was need.

Case 4

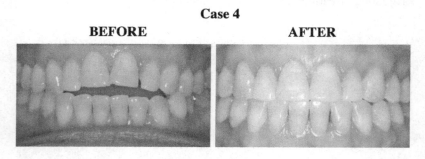

Case 5: Restorative and gum treatment was followed by orthodontic treatment. In addition to straightening teeth, here the purpose of

orthodontic treatment was to correct the back molars (upright), fix the patient's bite, and create enough space for two implants to fit properly.

Case 5

BEFORE   AFTER

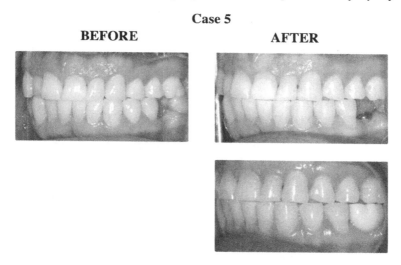

Cases 6, 7, 8 and 9: Restorative and gum treatment was followed by cosmetic treatment.

Case 6

BEFORE   AFTER

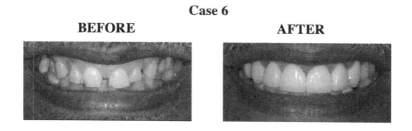

Case 7

BEFORE   AFTER

Case 8

BEFORE   AFTER

Case 9

BEFORE   AFTER

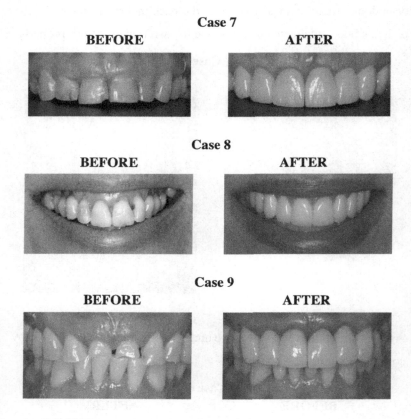

Made in the USA
Columbia, SC
21 September 2024

42077373R00055